# History of Nostril-Hair Removal:
# A Speculative Journey

*Collaborative effort by Chat-GPT
and Zeeshan Mahmud*

# Introduction

We've all had that moment. Maybe it's in the bathroom at a wedding, and you catch your reflection just right under that weird fluorescent lighting. You're looking sharp in the new suit, hair's perfectly in place, and just as you're about to give yourself a confident nod, you spot it: the rogue nose hair.

It's hanging out there like it's on vacation, waving at everyone who walks by, begging for attention. Suddenly, you're less James Bond and more *"Uncle Tony, who's kept his 'natural look' since '87."* You try the subtle "rub-and-check" maneuver, as if it's somehow going to tuck itself back in. No dice. And now you're panicking, searching for anything in your arsenal of toiletries—a pair of scissors, some nail clippers, heck, even a fork—to avoid walking out of there like the human version of Bigfoot.

Let's face it: at some point, we've all grappled with the age-old, nose-hair-fueled existential crisis. That stray, defiant hair has humbled kings, rattled CEOs, and reduced us all to mere mortals armed with tweezers and a silent prayer. And the funny thing is, while we all struggle with it in private, nostril hair removal has been a public affair for centuries. The saga of nose hair management—dating back to our woolly, prehistoric ancestors—is long, storied, and yes, occasionally downright absurd. Because when it comes to taming those tiny little whiskers, humans will apparently stop at nothing.

So, consider this your invitation to delve into the bizarre, brave, and occasionally terrifying history of nose hair removal. From ancient Egyptians to Victorian aristocrats, we'll uncover how each era tackled this unruly foliage in style. Or, well, in *some* kind of style. Prepare to laugh, wince, and maybe learn a thing or two. Because if there's one thing we can all agree on, it's that nose hairs don't discriminate. They're humanity's great equalizer—forever keeping us humble, one awkward bathroom encounter at a time.

# Chapter 1: When the First Homo Sapiens Took a Good, Hard Look in the Mirror

Let's rewind to when the human species first looked in reflective surfaces—possibly in a still pond or a really shiny rock—and thought, "Maybe I could do without the thicket growing from my nose." And just like that, the epic of nostril hair removal began. Sure, we might be tempted to imagine ancient humans as stoic survivalists too busy inventing fire and dodging saber-toothed tigers to think about their grooming habits. But you can't tell me that in a camp full of hunter-gatherers, no one ever leaned over to a friend and said, "You know, Grok, that nose hair might be a bit much."

Fast forward to the Ancient Egyptians, who—when they weren't too busy building enormous tombs and performing complex rituals on corpses—also pioneered personal hygiene trends. The Egyptians, masters of cosmetics and body grooming, believed nasal hair was like those TV antennas of the '80s that your dad refused to take down even though the signal was terrible. Egyptian priests, for instance, were known to pluck every single hair from their bodies to keep clean, and yes, that included nostrils. And while we can't confirm it, we'd like to think there was an Egyptian Jerry Seinfeld type going, "What's the deal with these nose hairs?"

Ancient Egypt was obsessed with cleanliness and appearance, and, yes, even nose hair was part of that. Egyptians considered body hair unclean and went to incredible lengths to keep themselves hair-free, including from those hard-to-reach nostrils.

## Ancient Egyptian Hygiene and Beauty

Ancient Egyptians believed in the power of grooming not just for beauty, but as a sign of purity and spiritual cleanliness. Priests especially had to be "pure" before performing any sacred rites, which meant they removed every visible hair from their bodies, including eyebrows, scalp, and, indeed, nasal hair. High-ranking officials and royalty had a preference for wigs, bald heads, and clean, smooth skin, which they achieved through various tools, oils, and primitive razors crafted from flint or copper.

Nose hair might have been seen as part of that pesky, unsightly "body hair" that needed regular attention. Egyptians didn't have our high-tech devices, so they used tweezers and other sharp instruments for plucking—tools often made of bronze or copper. There's even some evidence that ancient Egyptian grooming kits included small tweezers dedicated to hair removal, along with rudimentary razors and even beeswax for early depilatory efforts.

## Ancient Assyria and Babylon: Nasal Hair Lore?

As we trace nasal grooming further back, we find that other ancient civilizations also took hygiene and grooming seriously, though for slightly different reasons. In Assyria and Babylon, both cultures put a lot of emphasis on the head and facial hair, with beards especially having deep cultural importance. Babylonian and Assyrian men often wore long, carefully curled beards that symbolized status, masculinity, and authority. While there isn't direct evidence that they trimmed nose hair in the way the Egyptians did, it's likely that they maintained a close grooming regimen, possibly involving nasal hair management to keep their prized beards and faces looking neat.

In Assyrian and Babylonian cultures, cleanliness was associated with nobility and strength, so it's not hard to imagine that they, too, had some primitive practices for tackling nose hair. Tools for shaving and grooming have been found in archaeological digs, suggesting that grooming—including the subtle management of facial and nasal hair—was likely practiced by upper classes. Babylonian beauty routines may have also included scented oils to keep their curls glossy and their skin soft, meaning that they were hardly strangers to the grooming game.

## A Few Historical References

One of the earliest written hints about body grooming practices comes from Sumerian clay tablets dating back to around 4,000 BCE. While these don't specifically mention nose hair, they do detail bathing practices, oils, and combs, revealing that ancient Mesopotamian cultures cared deeply about appearance and hygiene.

In Egypt, we have references from the *Ebers Papyrus* (dating back to around 1550 BCE), which discusses body care and hygiene routines, though it doesn't specifically call out nasal hair. But a *British Museum* bronze mirror dating back to the 18th Dynasty (about 1550–1295 BCE) does showcase the Egyptians' obsession with reflective surfaces—proof of how integral grooming was to their daily life.

And it's hard to overstate the value Egyptians placed on tweezers. Archaeologists have found countless tweezers in tombs dating back to the Old Kingdom (c. 2686–2181 BCE), suggesting that some grooming tools were considered valuable enough to take to the afterlife.

---

### Evolutionary Origin of Nostril Hair

At first glance, those wiry nasal fibers seem like Mother Nature's idea of a practical joke, but in reality, they're a critical feature in our body's line of defense. Nose hair, or more scientifically, *vibrissae*, evolved to play a vital role in keeping us alive—think of them as the unsung heroes of the respiratory system.

**The *Why* of Nose Hair: A Frontline Defense**

Our noses are entry points for more than just oxygen. Every breath we take can bring in a cocktail of particles—dust, pollen, bacteria, viruses, and pollutants—all eager to get deeper into our respiratory system. Enter nose hair, which works like a physical sieve. The hairs capture these invaders before they reach the lungs, offering a first line of defense against harmful particles.

## A Double-Layer System: Nose Hair and Mucus

Nose hair operates in tandem with the mucus lining our nasal passages. Large particles get trapped by the hair, while smaller ones stick to the mucus, which contains antibodies and enzymes to help neutralize pathogens. The hair-mucus partnership effectively filters, captures, and neutralizes foreign particles in a synchronized defense system.

## The Evolutionary Benefits

1. **Protection Against Disease**: Ancient humans lived in environments with far more particulate matter than we do today. Between open fires, dusty plains, and living in close quarters with animals, they had constant exposure to pollutants and pathogens. Nose hair helped shield against respiratory infections by reducing the load of irritants and microbes entering the system.
2. **Moisture and Temperature Regulation**: Nose hairs also help to warm and moisten the air we breathe, creating a more lung-friendly climate. This ability would have been particularly beneficial in cold or dry climates, where warm, moist air protects the delicate tissue in our respiratory tract.
3. **Pheromones and Social Behavior**: Some evolutionary biologists speculate that nose hair may have contributed to early humans' sense of smell, indirectly aiding in social bonding and survival. Smelling pheromones and other scent markers helped humans identify kin, locate food, and detect threats. While nose hair isn't directly responsible for our sense of smell, its role in keeping the nasal passages clear likely supported scent detection, helping us navigate social cues critical to survival.

## Do We Still Need It?

In the modern world, where air filtration systems and purified indoor environments reduce our exposure to pollutants, nose hair might seem like it's becoming obsolete. But as any cold-weather jogger will tell you, that warming feature still proves its worth. Plus, as long as viruses and allergens exist, those little hairs continue to be our unsung first responders.

In the grand scheme of evolution, nose hair may be easy to overlook, but it's a testament to how even the tiniest adaptations serve crucial roles in keeping us thriving. And now, whenever you notice a rogue strand sneaking out, you can thank evolution for protecting you one sneeze at a time.

## Bringing It Together

So, while we may never know the exact moment a nose hair was first plucked in human history, one thing's clear: ancient civilizations knew that grooming was more than skin-deep—it was a pathway to purity, social standing, and even a sense of personal pride. Ancient Egyptians, and probably Assyrians and Babylonians, didn't just look in the mirror and see themselves; they saw a canvas for self-expression. And somewhere along the line, they probably noticed a stray nose hair or two… and did what any one of us would do: reached for the ancient equivalent of tweezers.

# Chapter 2: Romans and Greeks—Doing it for the Gods… or the Gladiators?

By the time the Greeks and Romans were running things, body grooming was full-on ritualistic. They saw a certain majesty in physical appearance—statuesque muscles, flowing togas, and clean nostrils to match. The Greeks had a particular fondness for what we now call "personal upkeep," and there's even some evidence of nasal hair plucking being part of the standard grooming routine. After all, if you were going to stand in a marble coliseum wearing nothing but a strategic strip of fabric, you wanted to look like a million drachmas.

In Rome, where gladiators were the influencers of the day, having a clean look was part of the gig. If you had nose hair, you might as well be wielding a wooden sword—no one would take you seriously. Roman barbers—tonsors—were your one-stop shop for head-to-toe (and yes, nose) grooming. And while they didn't have tweezers, they sure as Caesar had "volsellae," which were basically medieval torture tools for plucking hair. Imagine Dennis Miller narrating this: "Picture this, folks—Julius Caesar, conquering Gaul, but terrified of a pair of medieval tweezers like some kind of iron crab claw."

The Greeks and Romans had a famously intense relationship with grooming, hygiene, and… well, looking like marble sculptures. Now, it's worth noting that while body hair for men was seen as a symbol of virility, nose hair? Not so much. Both civilizations took nasal grooming quite seriously, and they had their fair share of quirky facts to keep things entertaining.

## Ancient Greece: The Birthplace of the Pinch-and-Pluck

The Greeks were trailblazers in philosophy, democracy, and — yes — grooming. You'd think that folks like Socrates and Plato would be too busy inventing Western thought to worry about nose hair, but no, even they had a grooming regimen. In fact, Greek men were known for their meticulous approach to body care, and nose hair removal was a matter of both hygiene and aesthetics.

Greek athletes, especially, were notorious for body hair removal. The Olympics weren't just about sports; they were about showcasing peak physical form, and any Greek competitor worth his weight in olive oil made sure there were no stray hairs to distract from his physique. Legend has it that Greek wrestlers even smeared themselves with olive oil before matches to prevent their opponents from grabbing onto their skin. So, you can bet they made sure that nose hairs were taken care of too; after all, a rogue nose hair could ruin even the most heroic of appearances.

## Enter the Tweezers: A Greek Grooming Staple

Ancient Greek grooming kits have been unearthed with — you guessed it — tweezers. Tweezers weren't just a handy accessory; they were considered an essential part of a respectable man's toolkit, right up there with strigils (those curious scraping tools used to remove dirt and oil from the skin). In fact, tweezers were so highly prized that many Greeks carried them around like a fashion statement, much the way some of us won't leave home without our smartphones. Wealthy Greek men were known to carry grooming kits in beautiful, small pouches or boxes made from ivory or precious metals. It wasn't uncommon to hear of wealthy Greek noblemen, after a hard day at the Agora, indulging in a nose-hair-plucking session with some fine bronze tweezers.

# History of Tweezers

Tweezer! An unassuming tool with a big historical footprint. Believe it or not, tweezers have been around nearly as long as humans have been grooming ourselves, and their story goes back to some of our earliest civilizations.

Tweezers — or at least their crude ancestors — date back to around 3000 BCE in Mesopotamia, which means we owe our thanks (and maybe a quick wince of empathy) to the ancient Sumerians. Archaeologists have unearthed some of the earliest examples of metal tweezers in what is now Iraq, often crafted from bronze or copper, suggesting that precision grooming had already become an art form.

By the time we get to ancient Egypt, tweezers were fully in vogue. Egyptians, who took their grooming rituals very seriously, were fond of plucking and shaving all sorts of body hair, considering smooth skin to be a mark of sophistication and cleanliness. They used tweezers made from copper — and in some cases, even gold. The Egyptians didn't just keep these tools for nose-hair duty either; tweezers were used to shape eyebrows, remove body hair, and, in some cases, prepare mummies. A true multitasker if there ever was one!

By the time tweezers reached ancient Greece, they'd become an everyday grooming essential for the well-to-do, especially among the upper echelons who saw personal grooming as a sign of sophistication. Some Greek tweezers were so well-designed and effective that you could probably still use them today (though the bronze might add a bit of a rustic touch to your kit). The Greeks even referenced tweezers in their art and literature, where keeping up appearances was almost a civic duty.

When the Romans got their hands on tweezers, they incorporated them into the *tonsor's* toolkit. Romans had a particular fondness for tools that could withstand a good deal of use — so Roman tweezers were generally durable, well-crafted, and even came in different sizes, proving that even 2,000 years ago, there was a "one for every need" philosophy in the grooming industry. Roman *tonsors* used tweezers alongside razors and mirrors in their bustling barbershops, where men gathered not only for a shave or pluck but also to swap the latest gossip.

Tweezers continued to evolve through the centuries, with each culture adding its own twist. In the Middle Ages, tweezers were a staple among European women, who would use them to pluck their hairlines to achieve that classic "high forehead" look that was the height of fashion. Fast forward to the Renaissance, and we start to see tweezers made from iron or steel, signaling an era when tools became as decorative as they were practical. By the time we reach the 17th century, tweezers were almost a luxury item — some even featured intricate engravings, monograms, or inlays of precious metals.

The modern tweezer we know and love (or hate, depending on your tolerance for pain) really came into its own during the 20th century. Inventors in the 1920s and '30s started designing tweezers with more precise tips, and they were soon marketed not just as a grooming tool but as a piece of essential equipment for tasks like surgery, electronics, and beauty. By the mid-20th century, the design was standardized, and tweezers had firmly established themselves as a tool we can't live without.

## Ancient Rome: Where Nasal Grooming Becomes an Art (and Maybe a Weapon?)

The Romans took Greek grooming practices and turned the dial up to eleven. Cleanliness was practically a state religion in Rome; they had public baths, regular shaving routines, and a borderline obsession with looking pristine. Nose hair, of course, was the enemy of any self-respecting Roman, especially since personal image was so closely tied to one's social rank. Roman men went so far as to ensure that even the hair in their noses was carefully pruned.

Enter *tonsors* — professional barbers who handled everything from beard trimming to nose-hair management. The *tonsor* was an important figure in Roman society, and his shop served as a kind of ancient salon-meets-gossip-hub. This was a place where business deals were struck, political debates waged, and — yes — the occasional stray nose hair obliterated. But let's not get carried away: plucking nose hair in ancient Rome wasn't exactly pleasant. Roman philosopher Seneca once joked that it was easier to face death than to face his tonsor wielding a pair of tweezers near his nostrils.

## Emperor Hadrian: The Hairy Outlier

Of course, there were exceptions to the rule. Emperor Hadrian, for example, was famous for his beard and full head of hair, a bold departure from the clean-shaven Roman emperors before him. Historians note that Hadrian embraced a more "natural" look in rebellion against the rigorous grooming practices of his predecessors. He may have been a proponent of facial hair, but let's not get carried away: it's doubtful he'd leave his nostrils unkempt, especially given the *tonsors'* intimidating precision.

## Pliny the Elder: Always Ready with Some Wisdom

Leave it to Pliny the Elder, Rome's favorite naturalist and "fact" collector, to have something to say about nose hair. In his *Naturalis Historia*, he rambles about the importance of grooming, noting that the Romans believed it helped in maintaining one's social status and personal cleanliness. Pliny, never shy with his opinions, made it clear that hair in odd places was not exactly Roman chic. Pliny may have been obsessed with medicinal plants and volcanic eruptions, but even he knew that nose hair had to be tamed.

## Roman Women and Nose Hair

While most of the evidence we have on nasal grooming is about men, let's not leave out Roman women. Women in ancient Rome had elaborate grooming routines of their own, and they were often as meticulous, if not more so, than their male counterparts. Wealthy women employed specialized slaves known as *ornatrices* who took care of all their grooming needs. These ladies of leisure may not have been as publicly worried about a stray nostril hair as their male counterparts, but let's face it — if Roman beauty standards were as unforgiving as they seemed, we can bet that nose hair wasn't left to flourish.

## Nose Hair Removal in Ancient Rome: Truly a Civic Duty

The Romans even had a saying, *"non curo, si sum niger, et nudus et crus hirsutus,"* which loosely translates to "I don't care if I'm dark, naked, and hairy-legged," emphasizing that *some* hair might be overlooked — but never nose hair. While being a bit rugged was acceptable, the nose was sacred ground, a frontier that simply had to be managed.

# Chapter 3: The Middle Ages and the Renaissance—When Nose Hairs Ran Wild (But Artists Kept Them Hidden)

With the Middle Ages, we hit the Dark Ages of nostril maintenance. Hygiene took a massive hit, probably because people were more concerned with not catching the plague than with their grooming habits. The church didn't help matters either, preaching that vanity was a sin. Yet, somehow, the painters and sculptors managed to depict patrons and nobility with nary a nose hair in sight. Michelangelo's *David* is flawless, right? No nose hairs peeking out, though I'd bet if David were real, he'd be the kind of guy who carries mini-scissors just for those occasional stray hairs.

During the Renaissance, folks began to turn back to the classics, embracing the Greek and Roman philosophies on beauty and form. Artists—who'd figured out how to make people look good with zero nostril intrusions—flocked to beauty secrets from yore, even if it involved Roman-style tweezers. And nose grooming made a quiet comeback among the elites who wanted to look noble and pristine—just in case Leonardo da Vinci showed up to paint them.

Nose grooming during the Middle Ages and the Renaissance wasn't exactly a hot topic at the local barbershop. For one, beauty and hygiene standards were worlds away from our modern concepts, and nose hair was probably more tolerated as part of life's natural gifts (even if less-than-ideal ones). But there are some intriguing historical hints about how people managed facial hair during these periods, and nose hair inevitably got caught up in the process!

In medieval Europe, hygiene was a bit of a rough-and-ready concept, especially during the earlier parts of the Middle Ages (around the 5th to 10th centuries). Bathing was sporadic at best, and dedicated nose grooming, as we know it, was minimal to nonexistent. Hair removal practices were often limited to the upper classes, who might occasionally use tweezers to shape their brows or remove stray facial hairs. While it's unlikely they used these tools specifically for nose hair, they were still aware of the social faux pas of an unruly face.

Medieval monks, on the other hand, sometimes practiced a kind of "hair asceticism" that involved trimming or shaving hair to maintain a humble appearance. Though mostly focused on head hair and beards, some fastidious monks may have paid attention to nose hair too — after all, they were already shaving patterns into their heads as an act of devotion.

When the Renaissance rolled around in the 14th century, everything changed. This was an era obsessed with refinement and appearance, especially among the Italian and French elite. Personal grooming became a cultural statement. Renaissance beauty was influenced by classical ideals, with a strong emphasis on facial symmetry and cleanliness.

People in the Renaissance began to understand hygiene better, and personal grooming took on a higher level of sophistication. While barbers were mostly concerned with shaving beards and trimming mustaches, they also performed all manner of facial "treatments," especially for wealthy patrons. These sessions likely included removing stray nose hairs, either with a trim or a careful tweeze. In Italy, where nose hair would disrupt the refined "Roman" profile that artists like Michelangelo were obsessed with, it's easy to imagine that barbers knew how to help clients handle any stray hairs.

There's no record of Leonardo da Vinci or Michelangelo pausing between masterpieces to pluck their nose hairs — although knowing da Vinci's fascination with anatomy, he might have sketched some if he had a tweezer in hand. Renaissance courts were also all about personal presentation, and courtiers would go to significant lengths to stay fashionable, which probably included some form of facial grooming.

The irony? The Renaissance men and women who had access to barbers and tweezers were grooming in candle-lit rooms with mirrors that offered only vague reflections. Even if they had the means, they didn't exactly have the tools to guarantee success in the nose-hair department!

By the end of the Renaissance, with grooming taking on such an elevated social importance, nose hair was likely on its way to being seen as something to "manage." This mindset would evolve into the "clean-shaven" expectations of later centuries, eventually leading us to modern-day nose hair trimmers and countless beauty guides on the art of facial grooming.

In short, while nose grooming wasn't always front and center during these eras, it was certainly lurking around the corners of medieval monasteries, bustling Renaissance barbershops, and in the reflections of countless dimly-lit mirrors!

# Chapter 4: Victorian Times—When Nasal Grooming Went Undercover (Literally)

Now, if you think today's obsession with "manscaping" is intense, meet the Victorians, who took personal upkeep to the extreme. Victorian etiquette books advised men and women to be well-groomed, and they meant *everywhere*. However, discussing body hair removal—especially nose hair—was akin to discussing unmentionables. They had an unwritten rule: "Keep it hidden and keep it clean." Meanwhile, doctors were developing terrifying contraptions resembling corkscrews to "cure" people with stubborn nasal hair issues. These devices were actually sold in catalogs like a bizarre mix between a health tool and a medieval device—because, you know, nothing says 'classy' like twisting a metal spiral up your nostril.

Victorian times — the era of strict etiquette, elaborate fashion, and grooming standards so intense that even nose hair couldn't escape the crosshairs of scrutiny. By the time we hit the Victorian age (1837-1901), society's collective obsession with cleanliness and orderliness had hit peak levels. Victorians didn't just want to look respectable; they wanted to appear as if they had their entire lives (and body hair) meticulously managed.

With the advent of indoor plumbing, improved lighting, and more refined grooming tools, personal hygiene became not just a daily ritual but practically a moral obligation. Cleanliness was associated with virtue, while an unkempt appearance was seen as evidence of moral failure. Victorians were practically fanatical about cleanliness, going so far as to invent items like *nose hair scissors* — yes, they were among the first to give us tools specifically designed to target those stubborn little intruders.

There were manuals dedicated to grooming etiquette, and they emphasized every aspect of personal hygiene, including nose hair.

These etiquette guides had strict rules on what was deemed acceptable, with advice on how gentlemen should handle the "unsightly" problem of nose hair. If you could see it, it was a problem — and if you were a well-to-do Victorian, it was your duty to take care of it.

The Victorian era also saw the barbershop flourish as a social institution, where men gathered not only to get a haircut and shave but also to undergo a rigorous grooming routine. Barbering evolved to include treatments like "singing" (yes, they would use a small flame to singe off any stray facial hairs). But for those who preferred precision over pyrotechnics, the barber's kit also contained miniature scissors, often silver-plated or ornately engraved, that were used for trimming nose hair.

Victorian barbers knew they had to be subtle. After all, nose hair might be an embarrassing topic for a gentleman to raise. So the barber would casually "take care of it" while trimming a mustache or beard, perhaps with the faintest of nods and no words exchanged. This was the birth of the unspoken social contract that still persists today in barbershops: nose hair is handled, no need to bring it up.

Victorian women were often expected to go above and beyond in their grooming — elaborate routines that could take hours. However, women's grooming tools were mostly geared toward eyebrow shaping and facial hair, as nose hair trimming was considered more of a masculine endeavor. But that didn't mean they were exempt from the expectations of a flawlessly groomed appearance.

In fact, some Victorian women took matters into their own hands with at-home "hair removers." The advertisements of the time are legendary: tinctures, waxes, and even highly questionable chemical mixtures were marketed to Victorian ladies for hair removal — although nose hair is one area they probably didn't risk putting mystery chemicals!

The Victorian obsession with propriety didn't stop at the masses; even high society had its grooming rituals scrutinized. Prince Albert, Queen Victoria's husband, was known for his impeccable grooming. While there are no direct accounts of Albert's nose hair routine, you can bet that a man who sported the polished, aristocratic look of the time wouldn't have let a rogue nose hair sully his refined appearance. After all, the Queen was watching, and her standards were high!

Oscar Wilde, with his penchant for the dramatic and his meticulous style, would have surely been on top of such things too. Though better known for his wit than his grooming, Wilde's reputation as a dandy suggests he would have embraced the era's grooming standards, perhaps even delighting in the ritual of an extra meticulous trim.

By the end of the Victorian era, grooming had transformed into a kind of high-stakes social sport, with nose hair getting its due attention as part of the fastidious "rules" of appearance. The Victorians laid the groundwork for our modern grooming standards, treating personal hygiene as both a public duty and a reflection of one's moral character.

# Chapter 5: Nose Hair Trimming Across Cultures - A Global Tour of Follicular Finesse

Nose hair: the ultimate universal connector. It doesn't matter where you come from or which god you pray to—at some point, everyone has looked in the mirror, noticed those rogue nostril curls, and thought, *"Yeah, that's gotta go."* Across history, humans everywhere have taken various approaches to taming these nasal intruders, and the methods and beliefs vary as wildly as the local cuisine. Some cultures treat nose hair with a stiff upper lip and a trusty pair of scissors, while others elevate it to a full-blown ritual. Let's take a tour through history and geography to explore the diverse, and often surprising, world of nose hair grooming.

*Ancient India: Ayurvedic Attention*

India, the birthplace of yoga, meditation, and Ayurvedic medicine, was also home to some rather intricate grooming routines. Ayurveda, India's ancient wellness system, didn't just focus on balancing the body and mind; it was serious about bodily maintenance. According to Ayurvedic texts, nose hair trimming wasn't merely a matter of appearance but a way to balance *doshas* (bodily energies). Practitioners believed that proper grooming, including trimming unruly nose hairs, could improve breathing and reduce excess heat in the body. Nose hair maintenance was considered just as crucial as oil massages or nasal rinses, all part of a holistic self-care regimen.

*Ancient China: The Yin and Yang of Grooming*

In ancient China, grooming practices were closely tied to the principles of harmony, health, and longevity. According to traditional Chinese medicine, every part of the body plays a role in maintaining *qi*, or life force, which flows through the meridians. While Chinese medicine emphasized the protective role of nose hairs in filtering harmful elements, too much of a good thing—say, sprouting an unruly forest from your nostrils—was seen as disrupting one's natural balance.

Early Chinese texts don't go into specifics on nose hair trimming techniques, but historians believe that sophisticated grooming tools, such as small scissors and tweezers crafted from bronze, were used. Chinese nobles and scholars were known for their meticulously groomed appearances, and, just like in Ayurveda, removing excess nasal hair was considered a step toward maintaining health and inner harmony.

*Japan: The Art of "Nostril Consciousness"*

Fast forward a few centuries to Japan, where grooming evolved into an art form, with specific rituals for almost every aspect of personal care. In the Edo period (1603–1868), samurai and courtiers prided themselves on immaculate appearances. Known for their high-top knots and perfectly shaved faces, samurai would never leave nose hair unkempt. Japanese grooming tools became so precise that craftsmen made tiny scissors specifically designed for delicate tasks like trimming nasal hair without causing irritation or injury.

However, Japanese culture also embraced the philosophy of *wabi-sabi*—the beauty of imperfection. A little bit of natural fuzz was okay, as long as it was subtle. Thus, "nostril consciousness" became a balancing act of removing excess hair while preserving a natural look. Essentially, a Japanese samurai could trim his nose hair and still uphold his bushido code, all while keeping his nostrils refined yet respectful.

*The Middle East: A Grooming Tradition Passed Down*

In the Middle East, grooming has long been associated with purity and personal pride. Historically, Arabic texts frequently discuss cleanliness as part of Islamic teachings, and grooming was a natural extension of this. Ancient Arab physicians like Al-Razi wrote about the health benefits of maintaining body and facial hair, including nose hair. Grooming rituals were often quite involved, with men trimming their beards, mustaches, and yes—nose hair—using small metal scissors or, if they were particularly daring, fire for singeing. Singeing was seen as a way to quickly and effectively manage unwanted hair, though it required a very steady hand (and possibly a prayer or two for safety).

To this day, you'll find Middle Eastern barbers offering "threading" and other traditional grooming methods, some even including a quick and efficient nose-hair trimming as part of the process.

*Indigenous America: The Balance of Nature and Hygiene*

Native American grooming practices varied greatly among tribes, but one recurring theme was respect for natural elements and an emphasis on cleanliness. While detailed records on nose hair removal specifically are sparse, personal grooming was commonly integrated into tribal practices. In tribes with warmer climates, where dust and dirt posed daily challenges, nose hair might have been more useful intact for its filtering abilities.

In contrast, some tribes likely practiced hair removal with tools crafted from bones or shells. To Native Americans, body grooming was a way to honor oneself and stay connected with nature. So, while nose hair may not have been meticulously managed in the way we might envision today, personal cleanliness was definitely prioritized.

*European Renaissance: When Grooming Meant Business*

We touched on this in earlier chapters, but it bears repeating: the Renaissance was a watershed era for grooming standards in Europe. The rise of the barbershop in Italy, France, and England gave people a new place to focus on their facial grooming, including nose hair. Although it was considered slightly uncouth to bring up nose hair at all, you can bet that aristocrats and nobles found discreet ways to manage it. European barbers of the time had everything from miniature scissors to specialized razors that could be used on small areas, so if you had the means, you didn't have to suffer with untamed nasal hair.

It was also during this period that the idea of public grooming standards really took off. In fact, barbers in Renaissance Italy were known for their flamboyant styles, with techniques for trimming everything from mustaches to stray hairs in odd places. If Michelangelo and his buddies had nose hairs peeking out, you'd better believe they were promptly snipped.

*Africa: Diverse Approaches to Grooming*

Africa's rich diversity of cultures and climates has led to equally diverse grooming practices. From the elaborate beauty rituals of ancient Egypt (where they invented tweezers, no less!) to the more minimalist approaches in Sub-Saharan tribes, grooming practices varied widely. In regions where dust was a constant nuisance, people may have found a certain benefit in letting nose hairs grow, embracing their role as tiny, natural dust-filters.

In North Africa, especially in areas influenced by ancient Egypt and later Islamic traditions, men and women embraced personal grooming as a part of daily life. Small scissors were often used to maintain facial hair, and local barbers would include nose hair trimming in their services if requested. The same care and pride in appearance that extended to their hair, skin, and nails naturally included their noses.


From fire-wielding Arab barbers to Renaissance Italians discreetly snipping in candle-lit salons, nose hair removal has taken on countless forms across cultures and epochs. What connects all these practices is the underlying universal desire to look good—or at the very least, to avoid awkward moments in candlelight or sunlight, when those wiry hairs catch a little too much attention. Each culture found its own way to grapple with those persistent strands, blending health, spirituality, and aesthetics into a unique approach that reflects its values.

# Chapter 6: Modern Times—Pluck It, Trim It, or Laser It, Just Don't Let it Show

And here we are in the modern era, where nose hair removal has become an industry in its own right. We've gone from simple plucking to trimming devices that look like tiny lightsabers. There's even nose waxing now—for people who laugh in the face of pain and love a good viral TikTok moment. Thanks to technology, we now have gadgets that target individual nose hairs, with laser precision, so we can look our best even if no one's close enough to notice.

And we've come full circle, my friend. From ancient Greeks to Instagram influencers, from a single reflective puddle to a whole aisle in CVS dedicated to trimmers, nose hair grooming has always been about one thing: asserting our superiority over nature, one stubborn follicle at a time.

**Appendix: Tools used in nose-hair removal**

The removal of nose hair may not seem like a pressing historical concern, but across cultures and centuries, people have found increasingly inventive tools to tame those pesky nostril intruders. Here's a whirlwind tour of nose-hair trimming methods that are as varied as the cultures that used them:

# 1. Ancient Egypt: Bronze Tweezers and Honey Mixtures

- The ancient Egyptians, renowned for their love of cleanliness and personal grooming, are believed to have crafted the first dedicated tweezers around 3000 BCE. Though these bronze tools were used for a range of purposes, Egyptian nobles and priests likely put them to work on rogue nose hairs, especially since nose grooming was essential to their ideas of beauty and hygiene.
- Fun fact: Egyptians were also big on depilation. For those particularly intent on smooth nasal passages, a paste made from honey and resin (a primitive version of waxing) may have been used to yank out those stubborn hairs.

# 2. Ancient India: Ayurvedic "Threading" Techniques

- In ancient India, Ayurvedic practices recommended threading for facial hair, which would sometimes extend to nose hairs. Skilled practitioners would twist threads to grip and pull out hairs in one quick motion. It wasn't for the faint of heart, but it was effective, especially as a technique in temples where appearance was part of spiritual cleanliness.

## 3. China's Han Dynasty (206 BCE – 220 CE): The Early Clippers

- During the Han Dynasty, Chinese inventors experimented with primitive scissors and clippers, often made from bronze, which could have doubled for basic nasal grooming. This was practical but still sharp enough to keep the tool work limited to professionals or brave souls willing to take on the risk.
- Later on, the development of metalworking allowed for sharper, more precise tools, which became popular grooming items among the nobility, particularly those close to the emperor.

## 4. Roman Empire: Tweezers, "Scalpellum," and the Skilled Barber

- Romans took nose-hair grooming seriously—mostly to avoid looking too rustic. Wealthy Romans and soldiers carried tweezers in their grooming kits (alongside other items like the *strigil*, a scraper for dirt and sweat). A sharp blade known as a *scalpellum* was also used by barbers to remove stubborn hairs; it was precise but required a practiced hand.
- Roman generals often traveled with their own barbers to ensure a "polished" look for important state meetings, and nose-hair maintenance was just as much a part of the routine as trimming beards and hair.

## 5. The Middle Ages in Europe: Goose Grease and Candle Wax

- While medieval Europe didn't have specialized nose-hair tools, makeshift methods emerged. Goose grease (a thick animal fat) was used to stick and remove unwanted nasal hair. For the bold, dripping wax from candles became a common, if painful, DIY method; once the wax dried around the hairs, a quick yank would pull them out. This was mostly done by peasants who didn't have access to professional barbers.

## 6. The Ottoman Empire: Curved Scissors and Hammam Barbers

- In the Ottoman Empire, a culture that prized grooming, hammam (bathhouse) barbers offered specialized curved scissors for nose-hair trimming. These were safer, allowing the barber to trim around the sensitive inner nostril without nicking the skin. Ottoman barbers were trained in this skill, and men in high society considered it a necessary step in regular grooming.

## 7. Japan's Edo Period (1603–1868): Bamboo Tweezers and Miniature Scissors

- Japanese samurai and courtiers of the Edo period carried compact grooming kits featuring bamboo tweezers or miniature scissors, which could be used for plucking or trimming nose hair. Samurai considered grooming a form of discipline, and nose-hair management was part of that ritual—ensuring that no stray hair would bring dishonor by sticking out during formal ceremonies.

## 8. Victorian Britain: The Debut of Personal Grooming Kits

- During the Victorian era, nose-hair trimming gained prominence in men's grooming kits, which featured ornate scissors with tiny, rounded blades specifically designed for safe nasal grooming. Victorian men became increasingly fastidious about grooming as they moved through crowded, smoke-filled cities, where nose hair became both a hygiene tool and, at times, a social liability.

## 9. Early 20th Century: The Electric Nose Trimmer

- The industrial age brought with it mechanized grooming. In the 1920s, electric razors were followed by early nose-hair trimmers with battery-operated mechanisms, providing a painless option for nasal maintenance. These trimmers became especially popular after World War II, as returning soldiers looked for ways to maintain the clean-cut look that had been enforced during their service.

Throughout history, nostril hair removal may have evolved from a spiritual duty to a social expectation, but it's clear that across time and culture, the desire for a clean nostril has remained remarkably consistent